MY STAY IN

Hospital

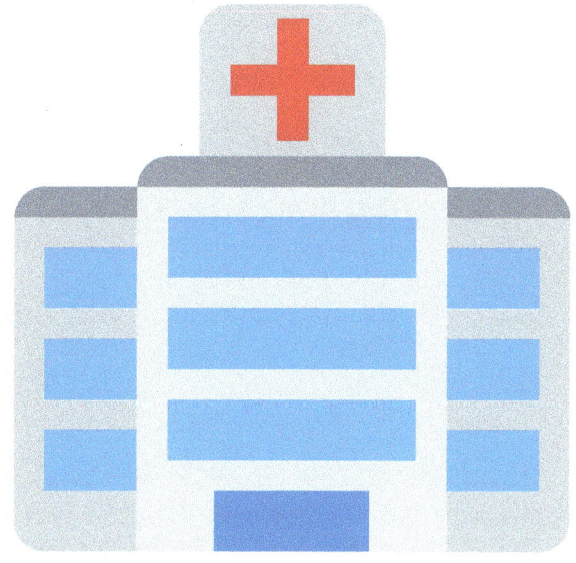

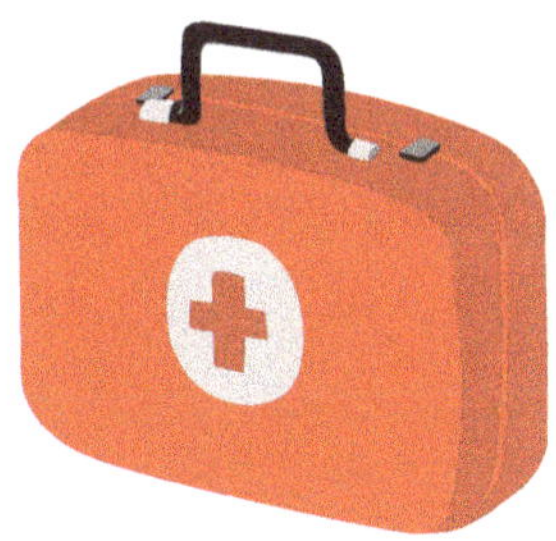

My Name: _______________________________

My Age: _______________________________

Hospital Name:

My Doctor's Name:

Reason for my Stay: 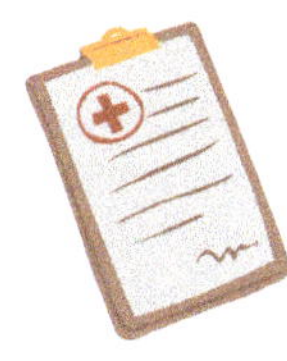

My Ward Name:

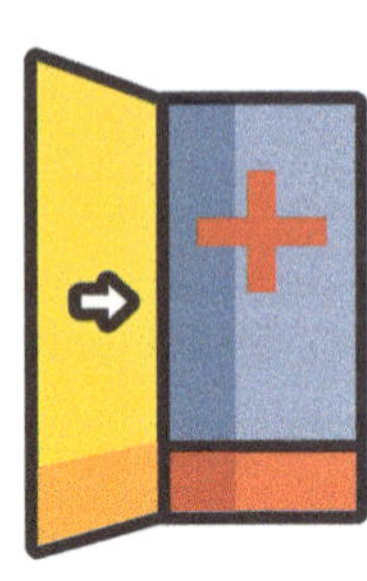

Room Number:

Nurses Names :

Hospital Staff:

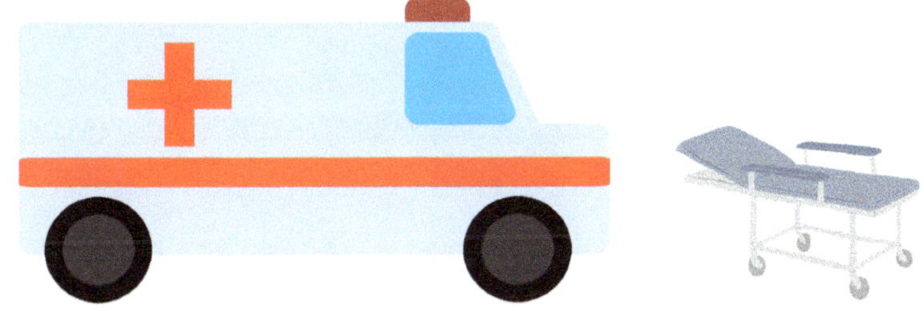

I arrived at Hospital by ...

____

____

____

____

My first impression of Hospital ...

____

____

____

____

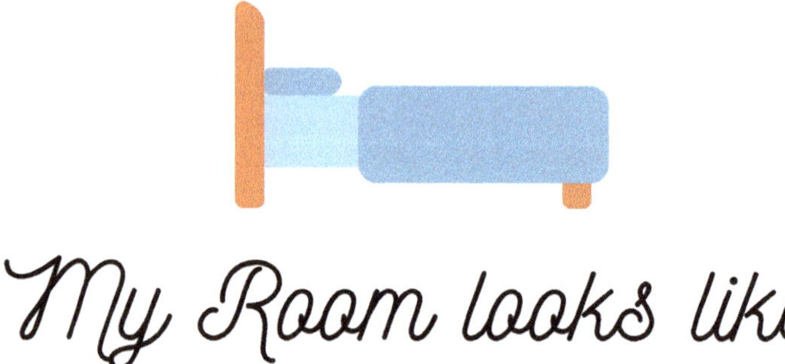

My Room looks like:

My favorite comforts:

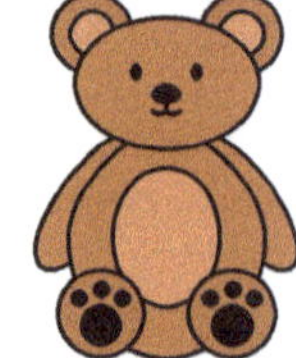

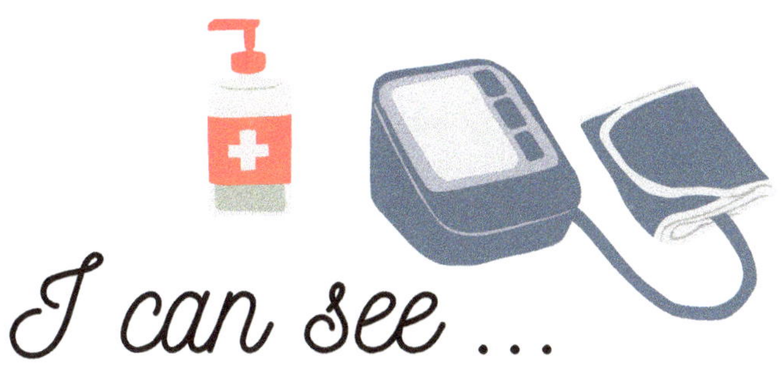

I can see ...

I am feeling.....

Drawing

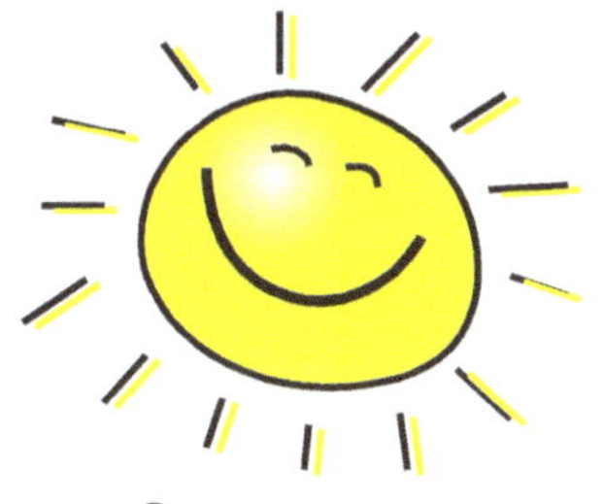

I look forward to ...

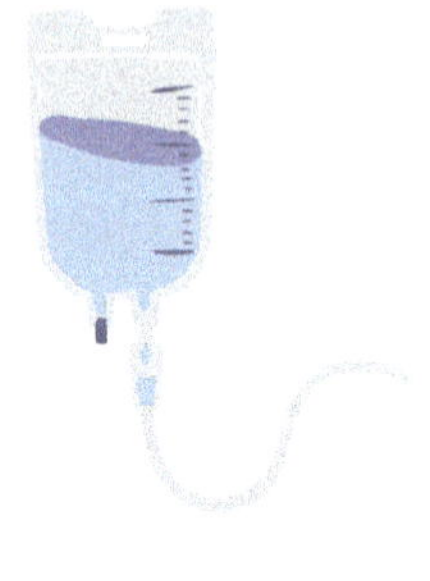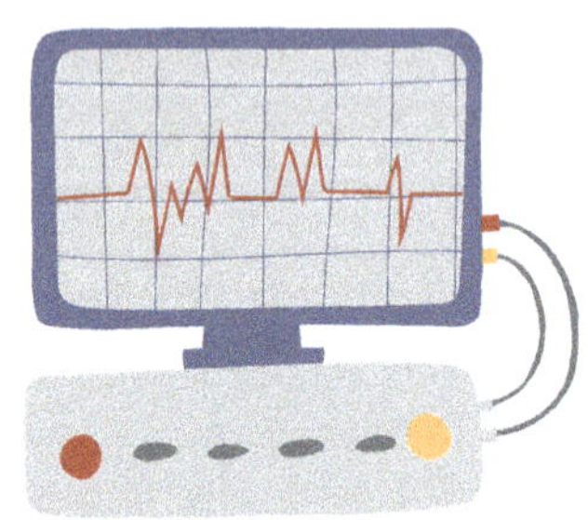

A question I would like to ask is ...

I would like to know this becuase ...

My favorite food in Hospital is:

My Breakfast Menu:

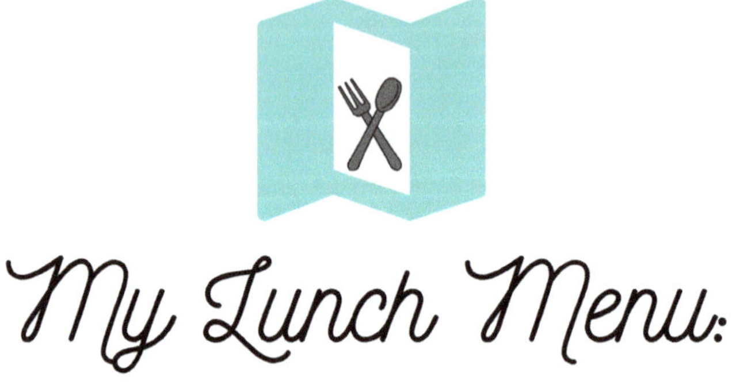

My Lunch Menu:

____

____

____

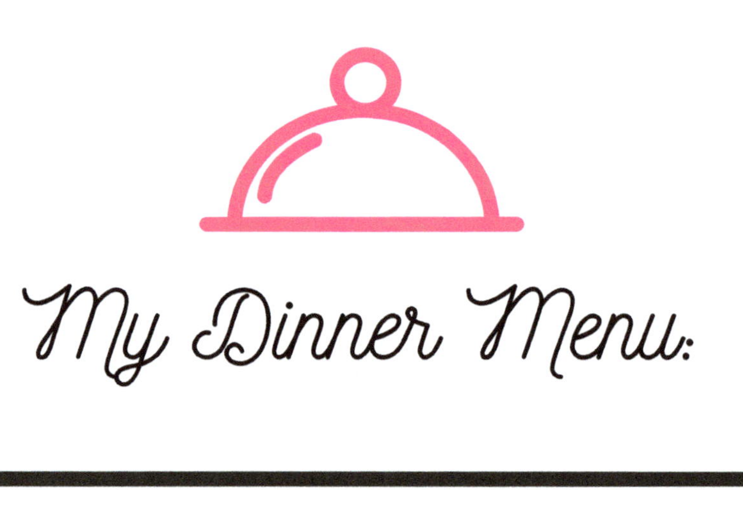

My Dinner Menu:

____

____

____

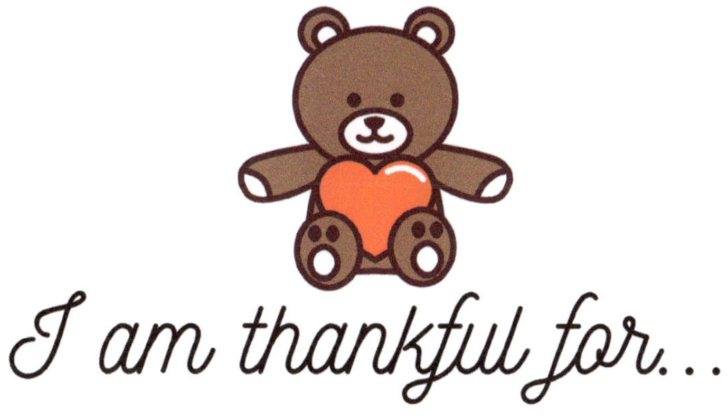

I am thankful for...

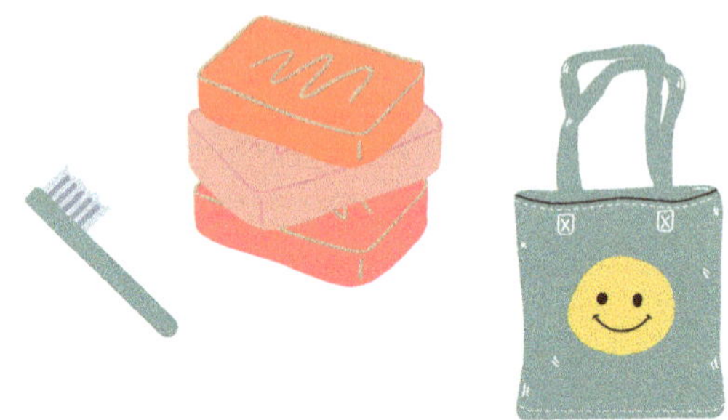

I would tell someone who is coming to this hospital ...

I spend my time in Hospital...

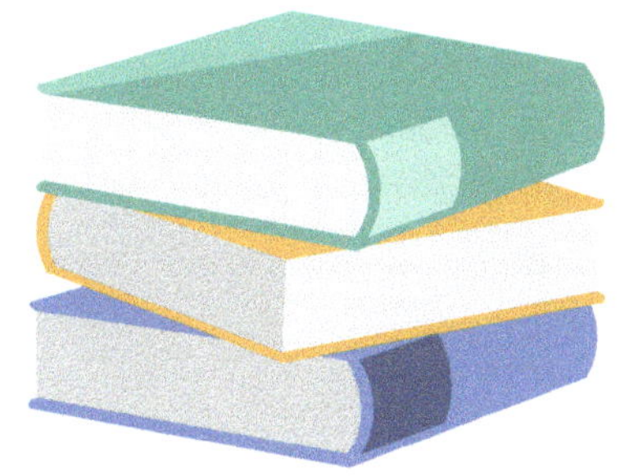

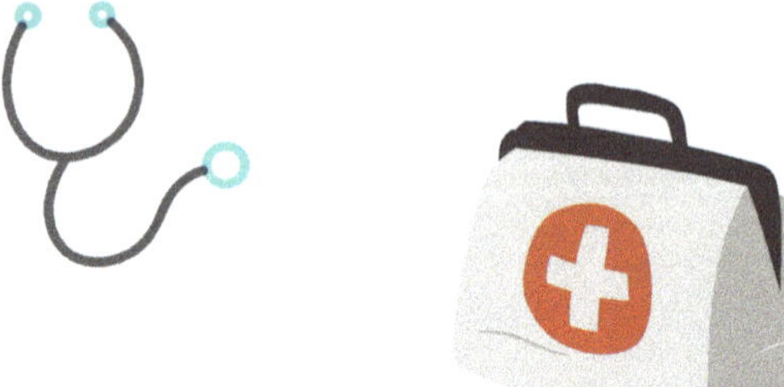

My Doctor tells me what to expect...

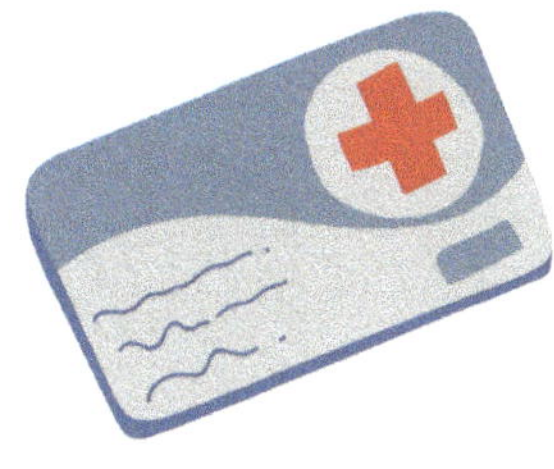

I would like to remember...

Something I have learnt while in Hospital …

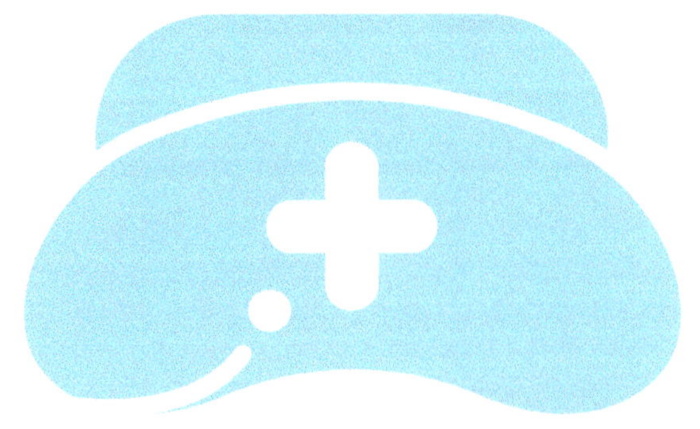

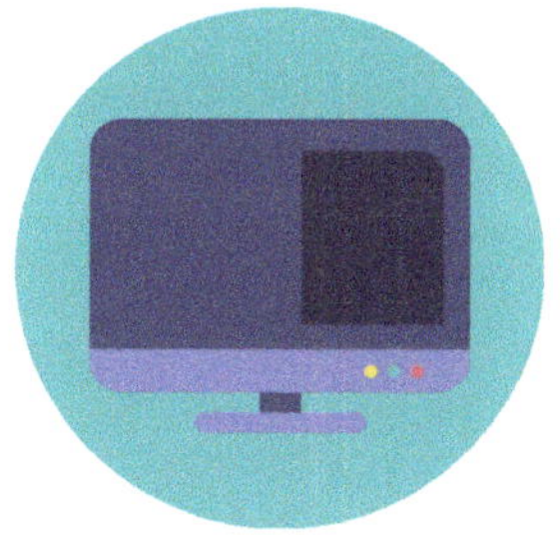

My entertainment system has ...

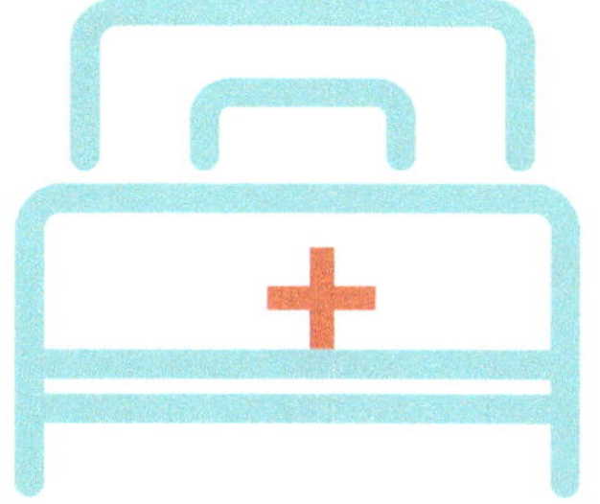

I would like to write about ...

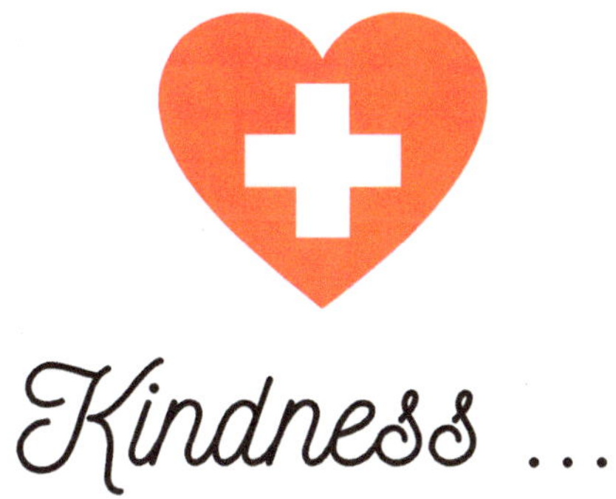

Kindness ...

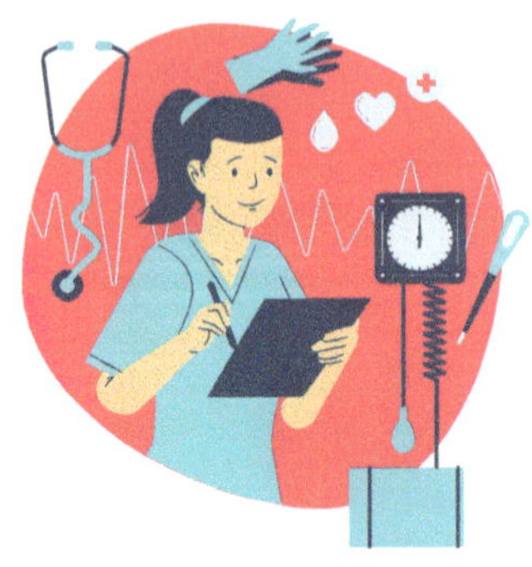

Something that surprised me about Hospital...

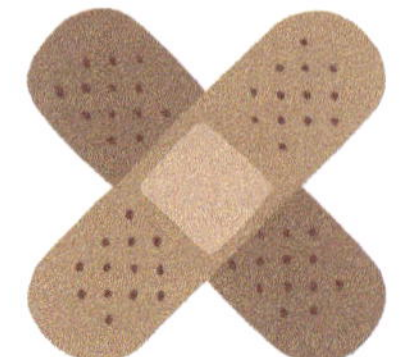

My Visitors ...

Autographs

Autographs

Favorite Keepsakes

Favorite Keepsakes

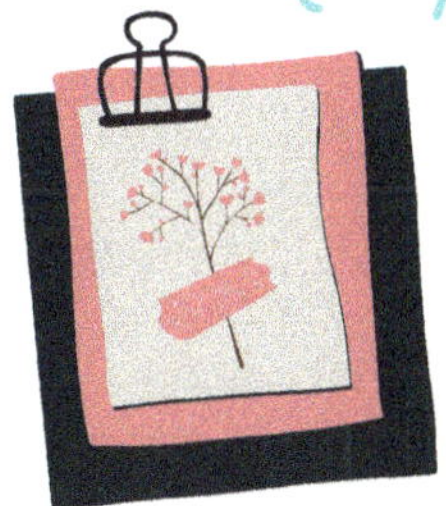

www.ingramcontent.com/pod-product-compliance
Lightning Source LLC
Chambersburg PA
CBHW040905070726
47599CB00038B/2317